50 THINGS TO KNOW ABOUT MAJORING IN PSYCHOLOGY

Tips for Success in College & Beyond

Alora Rands

50 Things to Know About Majoring in Psychology
Copyright © 2021 by CZYK Publishing LLC.
All Rights Reserved.
All rights reserved. No part of this book may be reproduced in any form or by any electronic or mechanical means including information storage and retrieval systems, without permission in writing from the author. The only exception is by a reviewer, who may quote short excerpts in a review.
The statements in this book are of the authors and may not be the views of CZYK Publishing or 50 Things to Know.

Cover designed by: Ivana Stamnkovic
Cover Image:
https://pixabay.com/photos/search/psychologist/

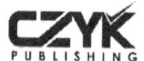

CZYK Publishing Since 2011.
CZYKPublishing.com
50 Things to Know

Lock Haven, PA
All rights reserved.

ISBN: 9798738703621

50 THINGS TO KNOW ABOUT MAJORING IN PSYCHOLOGY

BOOK DESCRIPTION

Are you thinking about getting a degree in psychology? Have you ever wondered what you can do with a psychology degree? Or maybe you want to know more about what to expect to learn while you work towards your psychology degree. If you answered yes to any of these questions then this book is for you. For every possible question you may have about a psychology degree, this book with have an answer.

50 Things to Know About Majoring in Psychology by author Alora Rands offers a approach to the psychology major that is more detailed than ever before. Most books on the psychology major will only cover the surface of what to expect as a psych major. Although there's nothing wrong with that, there are so many things to know about the psychology degree. Based on knowledge from the world's leading experts, you'll discover inside knowledge of how to succeed as a psychology major.

In these pages you'll discover the history of psychology, the jobs you can get with a psychology, tips for what you can expect during your college journey, and what you can expect after you get your degree. This book will help you decide if the psychology major is for you and give you tips to get ahead of your peers.

By the time you finish this book, you will know more about majoring in psychology than most college seniors, So grab YOUR copy today. You'll be glad you did.

TABLE OF CONTENTS

50 Things to Know
Book Series
Reviews from Readers
50 Things to Know About Majoring in Psychology
BOOK DESCRIPTION
TABLE OF CONTENTS
ABOUT THE AUTHOR
INTRODUCTION
ABOUT PSYCHOLOGY
1. THE BROAD AREAS OF PSYCHOLOGY
2. THE HISTORY OF PSYCHOLOGY
3. FREUD
4. PSYCHOLOGY IS A SCIENCE
5. PSYCHOLOGY IS GROWING
THE STUDY OF PSYCHOLOGY
6. HOW LONG IT TAKES TO GET A PSYCH DEGREE
7. HOW TO CHOOSE A UNIVERSITY
8. THERE'S A DIFFERENCE BETWEEN A BA AND A BS
9. WHAT YOU'LL STUDY
10. YOU'LL TAKE CLASSES OTHER THAN PSYCHOLOGY
11. YOU'LL HAVE TO DO MATH

12. PSYCH IS ONE OF THE MOST POPULAR MAJORS
13. CLASSES CAN BE VIRTUAL OR IN-PERSON

JOBS IN THE PSYCH FIELD
14. THE WORLD NEEDS PSYCH PEOPLE
15. THERE ARE JOBS IN PSYCH OTHER THAN BEING A COUNSELOR
16. BE PREPARED TO GET AN ADVANCED DEGREE
17. HOW MUCH PSYCHS ARE PAID
18. THE DIFFERENCE BETWEEN A PSYCHOLOGIST AND A PSYCHIATRIST
19. WHAT JOBS YOU CAN GET AFTER AN ASSOCIATE DEGREE
20. WHAT JOBS YOU CAN GET AFTER A BACHELOR'S DEGREE
21. WHAT JOBS YOU CAN GET AFTER A MASTER'S DEGREE
22. WHAT JOBS YOU CAN GET AFTER A DOCTORATE DEGREE
23. FIND YOUR NICHE

TIPS FOR STUDYING PSYCHOLOGY AND OTHER THINGS YOU'LL ENCOUNTER
24. STRENGTHS-BASED LANGAUGE
25. PEOPLE WILL ASK IF YOU CAN READ THEIR MINDS

26. YOU'LL DO A LOT OF WRITING
27. YOU DON'T ALWAYS NEED THE TEXTBOOK
28. GET INTO RESEARCH
29. SHADOW, SHADOW, SHADOW.
30. GET TO KNOW YOUR PROFESSORS
31. WORK ON CAMPUS
32. JOIN PSYCHOLOGY CLUBS
33. YOU CAN MINOR IN OTHER AREAS
34. YOUR MENTAL HEALTH MATTERS
35. YOU'LL READ A LOT
36. STUDY ABROAD
37. JOIN PROFESSIONAL ORGANIZATIONS
38. LEARNING BEYOND THE CLASSROOM: GET AN INTERNSHIP

PSYCHOLOGY SKILLS AND MORE

39. REFLECTION IS KEY TO THE PSYCH DEGREE
40. THE IMPORTANCE OF COUNSELING MICRO SKILLS
41. "TELL ME MORE"
42. ACCEPT CONSTRUCTIVE CRITICISM
43. GET ALONG WITH OTHERS
44. PSYCH JOBS ARE NOT EASY
45. PERSONAL GROWTH

AFTER YOUR DEGREE

46. YOU CAN ONLY BE LICENSED WITH A GRADUATE DEGREE
47. LICENSES DON'T ALWAYS TRANSER FROM STATE TO STATE
48. SEPARATE WORK FROM HOME
49. YOU CAN SPECIALIZE
50. BE YOUR OWN BOSS
FINAL THOUGHTS
Other Resources:
Other Helpful Resources
50 Things to Know

ABOUT THE AUTHOR

Alora Rands received her Bachelor of Arts in Psychology from the College of St. Scholastica and her Master of Arts in Child, Family, and School Psychology from the University of Denver. She is currently working towards her doctorate in School Psychology at the University of Minnesota, Mankato. She has been studying psychology for nearly 10 years and has worked as a psychology research assistant, statistics teaching assistant, and has been part of several research teams regarding the school-to-prison pipeline and equity in the school system.

Her research interests include developing interventions to target chronic absenteeism in the education system, social-emotional education for young learners, and the implementation of a successful PBiS or RTI system in the schools. When she is not researching, writing, or working on her degree, Alora is working with students who have reading disabilities or supporting youth who struggle with time management.

For more of her work, you can find Alora Rands on Vocal at https://vocal.media/authors/alora-r.

INTRODUCTION

*"You know too much psychology
when you can't get made because
you understand everyone's reasons
for doing everything"*

–Via (The Middle Journal)

HOW TO USE THIS BOOK

If you've purchased this book, odds are you've heard of the field of psychology and are trying to figure out if this path is right for you. Maybe you've always been interested in helping people and have already decided on psychology as your major. Or, maybe you're like me and started off as a biology major but at the first sight of blood in the cadaver lab, decided that you need to make a change ASAP.

Needless to say, you can use this guide to the psychology major whether you're a high school student researching majors for the first time, a college freshman trying to choose your path, halfway through your college career and need to make a change, or coming back to school to get a degree in your area of passion.

The field of psychology can lead to many rewarding and exciting careers. Because the discipline is so broad, you can either follow a designated career path, such as counseling, research, or social work, or pave your own career path and become a private practitioner of your own practice.

As someone who is first getting to know psychology, there's a lot to learn and so much to know. But where do you start? Instead of scouring the internet for various blogs that can tell you why you should choose a psychology major, use this book as your comprehensive guide to psychology as a discipline.

Not only will you learn the basics of psychology, but we'll go through the history of psychology, tips for college success, how to find your career focus, and even what you should know as you enter your career as a future psychology professional.

As someone who started off her career as a biology major and made the switch to psychology, I have a lot of experience in the area of psychology majors. Additionally, I have graduated with my Master of Arts in School Psychology and am currently pursuing my doctorate in the same discipline. For you readers, I hope to share the tips and information I wish I had known about psychology before I began my career.

So without further ado, let's learn about the psychology major.

ABOUT PSYCHOLOGY

The first step to discovering whether psychology is right for you is to learn about how this field came to be. Did you know that psychology stemmed from philosophy? Or that psychology has grown exponentially over the last century? Maybe you've heard of Freud, the Father of Psychology, but do you know why we psych people call him that?

In this section, we'll explore the basics of psychology and how it came to be a science. We'll cover the broad areas of psychology, its history, and psychology today.

1. THE BROAD AREAS OF PSYCHOLOGY

While there are many areas of study in the psychology field, some of the more common areas include developmental, perception-cognition, biological psychology, quantitative and social-personality. Developmental psychology looks at the brain and how it changes over a lifetime. Developmental psychologists may study children, the theory of mind, thoughts, language, and emotions.

Those who study perception and cognition may study consciousness, learning, memory, and how humans perceive events. Biological psychology looks at how biology and mental functions are related. These psychologists may research behavior, sensory processes, and animal behavior. They may also look at brain structure and biological functions.

Quantitative psychologists are mainly concerned with data, research methods, and correlational studies. Finally, social and personality psychologists will look at how an individual interacts with the environment and often looks at culture and behavior. [1]

2. THE HISTORY OF PSYCHOLOGY

While the practice of clinical and counseling psychology did not become popular until 1945, humans have been interested in psychological concepts for hundreds if not thousands of years. Psychology has deep roots in philosophy, and Rene Descartes (1596-1650) is one philosopher who believed that the mind and body were separate but influence each other. Little did he know that this would be a question that would intrigue many psychologists in the centuries to come.

Phrenology is another study that influenced modern psychology. The study of phrenology looked at how personality was related to the shape of the skull. Phrenologists believed that certain areas and the structure of the skull related to someone's personality traits. While this has been proved to be false, it does indicate that researchers knew that the brain somehow related to an individual's emotions, feeling, and personality.

Three researchers were key in finally developing a study of psychology in the 1800s: Hermann von Helmholtz, Ernst Weber, and Gustav Theodor Fechne. These founders of psychology studied psychophysics, which looked at the interaction between human behavior, perception, and the environment.

Going forward to the late 1800s and early 1900s, we saw the development of Wundtian Psychology and Structuralism. Wilhelm Wundt was the first person to have a psychology lab and he was mainly interested in the study of consciousness. Structuralism stems off Wundtian Psychology and mainly looks at the structure of the brain and how it relates to consciousness.

Next, Functionalism became a big topic in psychological study, and William James, G. Stanley Hall, and James M. Cattell were the leading studies on human consciousness, behavior, and the function of each component of the brain. Then, John Watson introduced Behaviorism and we begin to see research studies that have observable factors. Watson wanted to make psychology observable and measurable, and thus psychology became even more of a science. Mostly interested in how the environment impacts behavior, Watson only looked at undisputable facts to support his research.

Finally, cognitive psychology was introduced and is currently a practice that is currently studied today. Cognitive psychology is mainly concerned with how mental processes work and is the most popular approach to experimental psychology in modern research. [12]

The above information is just a brief history of psychology. Other psychologists influenced the practice and the science of psychology, such as Freud. But with this brief history, you will have a general understanding of how psychology became a science.

3. FREUD

Sigmund Freud lived from 1856 to 1939 and is known as the founder of psychoanalysis, a method that is still used today and that has influenced many modern practices that treat mental illness. Freud is likely one of the most interesting influencers of psychology and is famous for his belief that our past events impact our future. Not to mention is obsession with sexual deviance, dreams, and unconscious desires.

While it is well known that past and childhood experiences shape our future, Freud's theories are not necessarily the most popular nowadays because of his psychosexual stages of development. In summary, Freud believed that women became mentally ill because they suppressed psychosexual needs and that children had to experience different psychosexual stages (oral, anal, phallic, latent, and genital) to become a normally functioning adult. If one of the needs wasn't met, then that person would remain stuck in that stage and experience problems later in life.

Freud is also the creator of a structural model of psychology that is still referenced today even if it is not widely supported by all. His model is an iceberg where the conscious mind is what we see, but the unconscious mind makes up a large part of our psyche and remains in the dark and unseen. The three parts, the Id, Ego, and Superego are constantly at odds trying to balance our animal instincts and human morality.

He also introduced the concept of defense mechanisms, such as repression, denial, and projection as a way to describe how people react to stressful life situations. While these may not pertain to his overall model, many of the ways to suppress emotions are still discussed today. [13]

4. PSYCHOLOGY IS A SCIENCE

Don't let anyone tell you it isn't, because those biology and chemistry majors like to say their science is more superior than psychology. They couldn't be more wrong.

You'll often hear the term, "data-driven" because every decision psychologists make depends on data from assessments, questionnaires, tests, interviews, and more. When psychologists make a decision, it's never random. They are always looking for data to support their course of treatment.

5. PSYCHOLOGY IS GROWING

With more and more jobs each year, psychology is a growing field. Not only are there more jobs, but research is continuing to uncover more information about the human brain and psychological functioning. If you're interested in research, you can go into positive psychology, organizational psychology, educational psychology, and much more. Many other fields are discovering the benefits of psychology and mental health practices. So, more disciplines are looking for people who have experience studying psychology.

THE STUDY OF PSYCHOLOGY

Now that you have a general history of psychology and a plethora of fun facts, it's time to learn what you'll experience as a psychology major. While most of the study of psychology will cover broad areas, many colleges and universities offer electives in different areas. Are you ready to learn everything and more about the psychology degree? With this section, you'll have all the knowledge you'll need to be an informed psychology student.

6. HOW LONG IT TAKES TO GET A PSYCH DEGREE

Typically, it takes about four years of full-time study to get a bachelor's degree in psychology. However, if you get an associate degree before you enrolled in a four-year program, you can speed up the time it takes to get your degree and may even be able to finish your degree in two years. This is the same for anyone coming in with previous college credits or credits from qualifying advanced high school courses, such as Advanced Placement (AP) or College in the Schools (CIS). Typically, you can apply your general education credits towards your psychology degree so that you come in with advanced standing.

If you take your classes on campus, you'll likely spend the entire four years working towards your degree. If you take online classes, however, some programs offer accelerated courses that allow you to get your degree faster. But these programs are usually meant for those who already have some college credit. You could also opt to take more credits and enroll in summer courses to get your degree faster, but this will greatly increase your course load and you may find yourself feeling burned out.

On the flip side, you can take a more relaxed approach to your college education and take fewer credits each semester or quarter. If you were to take just two classes each semester instead of the full 18 credits, for example, it may take longer for you to get your degree, but you'll have more time for work and family obligations.

So even though the average time it takes to get a bachelor's degree in psychology is about four years, you can potentially speed up or slow down the time it takes for you to get a degree depending on the number of credits you come in with and the number of credits you take each semester.

7. HOW TO CHOOSE A UNIVERSITY

Deciding which university to attend for your psychology is a major decision, so there are many factors you should consider when choosing a university. For starters, you'll want to check to make sure the university you're interested in offers a psychology degree. Luckily, many universities do have psychology programs, but you should make sure to check, just in case.

With so many programs offering online options, your first major decision may be to decide if you want to attend classes virtually or in-person. While an in-person course may better suit individual learning styles, online classes allow for a lot more flexibility in your schedule and tend to be cheaper.

Secondly, you'll want to see what experiences the psychology program offers. Are there opportunities for research? Does the university have study abroad experiences? Are there any interesting psychology electives? Can you get a minor or concentration in a different area (such as social work, sociology, child psychology, forensic psychology, etc.)? Are there teaching assistantships?

By evaluating the experiences offered by a given program, you'll be able to evaluate how well a program fits your needs. If you really want to study abroad but a university doesn't have the option, for example, you may want to choose a different school.

Additionally, you'll want to look at your program's options for financial aid, cost of tuition, opportunities for room and board, student organizations, school culture, student resources, and on-campus work. The moral of the story, when you're looking for a psychology program, you'll want to do a lot of research on the program and the school.

While you can find a good amount of information online, one of the best ways to get more information about a school is to talk to professors, current students, and academic advisors. Plus, you'll want to visit a school to see the campus and student life before you make your decision on any particular school.

8. THERE'S A DIFFERENCE BETWEEN A BA AND A BS

Do you want to get a Bachelor of Arts (BA) or a Bachelor of Science (BS)? Maybe you've heard of these two degrees, or maybe this is the first time you've heard that there's a difference between the two. First of all, not every program will offer both a BA and a BS. In fact, many universities will offer one or the other, but not both. And if you're me, you won't be aware of that until you receive your diploma and wonder how they decided to award you a BA.

The main difference between a Bachelor of Arts and a Bachelor of Science is research and science-based classes. With a BA, you'll take more humanities classes and take a more theoretical approach to psychology and its practice. But with a BS, you can expect more research-based classes. Now you may be thinking, is one better than the other?

Honestly, it does not matter if you get a BA or a BS in psychology. However, a BS may give you more research experience if you're interested in pursuing a career in psychological research and plan to go on to advanced study. But having a BA will not hurt your chances of getting into a graduate program. After all, you will still possess a comprehensive knowledge of psychology. If you're looking for proof, I have a BA in psychology and still experienced no issues getting into master's and doctorate level programs.

9. WHAT YOU'LL STUDY

One of the biggest questions you may have about the psych degree is about what classes you'll take. Typically, your coursework will cover psychology in a broad sense. You'll be exposed to the many areas of psychology and get more of a "jack of all trades but master of none" education, meaning you'll encounter numerous topics, but you won't become an expert until advanced programs.

While there is a standard set of classes that every credible psychology program is required to have in their degree program, other programs will offer electives that dive deeper into areas of specialization, such as forensic psychology, counseling psychology, personality, and human behavior. If you're interested in these types of courses, make sure to check out the courses that your program offers or talk to an academic advisor for more information.

However, here is a list of the most common classes you will encounter when working towards your psychology degree:
- History of Psychology
- Introduction to Psychology
- Introduction to Statistics
- Research Methods – Theory and Application

Additionally, other courses you may be able to take include:
- Abnormal Psychology
- Adolescent Psychology
- Adult Psychology
- Animal Behavior
- Child Psychology
- Human Cognition
- Neuroscience
- Personality Theory
- Psychology of Perception
- Social Psychology [2]

While this is in no way a comprehensive list of courses, it is a general list of the common topics you'll encounter in a bachelor's program. However, once you go on to more advanced studies, such as master's and doctorate, you'll find classes more focused on a specialization or area of interest.

10. YOU'LL TAKE CLASSES OTHER THAN PSYCHOLOGY

Quite honestly, things don't really get interesting until after your second year in school. For the most part, your first two years will be filled with liberal arts courses and prerequisites. Even if you declare your major early on, you'll still be required to take a certain number of credits in another area, such as history, art, or science.

However, if you come into a program with qualifying high school credits or college credits, you may be able to skip some of the general education courses. If you're interested in whether your school accepts credits, it's best to contact your advisor or a university recruiter to get more information on what they accept and what they don't accept.

11. YOU'LL HAVE TO DO MATH

A psych degree is not complete without courses in statistics. In your undergraduate program, you'll likely need to take only one or two sections of statistics. But in advanced graduate programs, there are several stats classes you'll have to endure. So, be prepared to do some math.

Granted, understanding statistics in psychology is incredibly important to the science. In fact, you'll need a basic understanding of statistics if you want to read research articles and understand the results of study. If a finding is significant, you'll need statistics to help you figure out the true implications of a research finding. If you are interested in doing your own research, you'll especially need to know statistics because you'll be expected to perform your own analyses.

While you will need to learn how to do the physical math and calculations (as with any math class), you'll also be introduced to the software that does the statistical calculations for you, such as SPSS. So yeah, you will need to do some math. But it will become automated once you learn the programs.

12. PSYCH IS ONE OF THE MOST POPULAR MAJORS

According to the National Center for Education Statistics, 6% of college students will choose the psychology major. This makes it the fourth most popular degree behind the business, social sciences, and education. [11]

Psychology is popular because the field itself is so interesting. New research is constantly being released and there are so many opportunities to be a part of it. Additionally, there are many different jobs you can get with a psychology degree. We will go over all of this information more in-depth later in this book.

13. CLASSES CAN BE VIRTUAL OR IN-PERSON

Because we live in a world where we can attend class in person or be present in an online format, many programs offer virtual classes. Depending on your learning style and preferences, this can be a good thing or a bad thing.

If you are someone who can manage their own time, is organized, and enjoys flexibility, then a virtual program may be right for you. Online programs definitely have their perks: you can work while in school, attend classes at night, and do your work when you please. But if time management is not your strength and you tend to procrastinate, then an online program may not be the best option. For those who prefer more interaction with their classmates and professors, then an in-person program may be your best choice.

JOBS IN THE PSYCH FIELD

Learning about what to expect as a psychology major is very important, but what about what you can actually do with a psychology degree? If you're interested in psychology, odds are you've been asked if you want to be a counselor. While the field of counseling is noble and exciting work, there is much more to learn about jobs in the psychology field.

14. THE WORLD NEEDS PSYCH PEOPLE

The psychology field has great job prospects. The Bureau of Labor Statistics states that psychology jobs will grow around 3% between 2019 and 2029, but the world will continue to need more psychology professionals. As more people become aware of the importance of mental health, more psychologists will be needed to work with them. If you go into social work, however, those jobs are growing at a rate of 13%, which is much faster than most jobs. So, job prospects in the helping field are excellent. [10]

15. THERE ARE JOBS IN PSYCH OTHER THAN BEING A COUNSELOR

Many people think that counseling is the only thing you can do with a psychology degree. However, there are so many options for other jobs. In fact, you can do just about anything with a psychology degree if you want to. While some people do go on to be counselors, others may work in marketing, corrections, or education. The opportunities are endless.

16. BE PREPARED TO GET AN ADVANCED DEGREE

In order to become licensed, you need to at least have a credible master's degree from a psychology program. Unfortunately, you cannot practice as a psychologist with just an associate or bachelor's degree. While there are jobs that you can get with these degrees (more on your options below), you will not be qualified to be a counselor or practicing psychologist until you have a master's or doctorate degree and pass a state licensing exam. So, be prepared to continue your study of psychology for at least two more years to get a master's degree.

17. HOW MUCH PSYCHS ARE PAID

According to the Bureau of Labor Statistics (BLS) [10], psychologists can make up to $80,370 each year. The salary, however, will depend on your level of education, experience, and where you live. Typically, those who have doctoral degrees will make the most, but those who have bachelor's degrees will be closer to $40,000 each year. For this reason, it's definitely encouraged to get an advanced degree.

18. THE DIFFERENCE BETWEEN A PSYCHOLOGIST AND A PSYCHIATRIST

While both psychologists and psychiatrists work to help those who suffer from mental illness, their positions are very different. Psychiatrists are licensed, medical doctors who will assess a client and prescribe medication to manage psychological symptoms, such as anxiety, depression, bipolar disorder, and more. They will also diagnose patients with mental disorders if they have the data and assessments to show significant results.

Psychologists, on the other hand, can diagnose patients with mental illnesses, but they will not prescribe medication. Instead, psychologists will develop treatment plans for their clients, perform counseling, and work with their clients to manage mental illness.

Additionally, psychiatrists need to become a doctor before specializing in psychiatry. It can take as much as twelve years to gain the qualifications to become a psychiatrist. However, a psychologist will likely have a master's or a doctorate degree that will take anywhere from two to six years to achieve depending on the program.

19. WHAT JOBS YOU CAN GET AFTER AN ASSOCIATE DEGREE

An associate degree is typically a two-year degree that allows you to get entry-level jobs in the psychology field, such as a youth counselor, administrative assistant, family advocate, mental health associate, or psychology aid. Most of the time, those who get an associate degree generally go on to get a bachelor's degree. [6]

20. WHAT JOBS YOU CAN GET AFTER A BACHELOR'S DEGREE

A bachelor's degree in psychology is a great steppingstone to become a psychology professional. Even though you cannot be a practicing counselor with a bachelor's degree, a bachelor's degree is often a prerequisite for advanced programs. With your bachelor's degree in psychology, you can become a police officer, caseworker, community worker, corrections officer, research assistant, psychiatric technician, and more. [7]

21. WHAT JOBS YOU CAN GET AFTER A MASTER'S DEGREE

With a master's degree, you have many more opportunities for careers in the field of psychology. Usually around two years in length, you can get a master's degree to become an organization/industrial psychologist, counseling psychologist, social psychologist, forensic psychologist, or school psychologist, to name a few. [8]

22. WHAT JOBS YOU CAN GET AFTER A DOCTORATE DEGREE

A doctorate degree is the highest level of degree that you can achieve in the field of psychology. While clinical psychology, research, and university-level teaching are all positions you can get with a doctorate degree, you may also become a human resource manager, educational psychologist, marketing director, or an administrator. You can also get doctoral degrees in your chosen field to become even more specialized and open your own private practice. [9]

23. FIND YOUR NICHE

Research, counseling, teaching, clinical, what to do? Most importantly in your psychology career, you should find your passion in psychology early in your career. While many people do make career changes late in life, it's best if you know what area of psychology you'd like to pursue. This is especially important if you want to reach the doctorate level because you'll want to get into research and teaching assistantships in your bachelor's program.

If you know you want to get a job out of undergrad and do not want to go for an advanced degree, participating in research or getting a teaching assistantship isn't necessary, but could be an added boost to your resume. But because most jobs in psychology require at least a master's degree, make sure you research your job options early so that you can work towards those positions by getting internships and other experiences.

TIPS FOR STUDYING PSYCHOLOGY AND OTHER THINGS YOU'LL ENCOUNTER

So how do you succeed as a psychology student? What are some tips and tricks that you should know when studying psychology? In this section, we'll explore all this and more, so you won't encounter any surprises as you navigate your psychology degree.

24. STRENGTHS-BASED LANGAUGE

In the psychology field, strengths-based language is the best way to discuss challenges with your clients. In psychology, you never want to speak negatively about a client to other professionals and especially to the client themselves. Instead, psychology professionals focus on the strengths of their clients, including positive characteristics, achievements, and progress made.

That being said, many psychological professionals also avoid labeling their clients. So instead of saying a client is an "addict," for example, you would refer to the client as, "__ suffers from addiction." That way, you are not talking about your client negatively and are referring to their challenge or mental illness as something that can be improved or treated.

If you avoid strengths-based language, you run the risk of forming a negative relationship with your client or their family, overlooking progress, or viewing your client as a disorder and not a person. For those reasons, get used to using strengths-based language.

25. PEOPLE WILL ASK IF YOU CAN READ THEIR MINDS

Mind reading would be the perfect skill as a psychologist, you wouldn't have to work nearly as hard to counsel your clients! But sadly, we're only human and can't read minds. While it may seem funny or like a joke, some people believe psychologists are mind readers. You'll be surprised by how many times you meet someone for the first time and after they learn you are studying psychology, they'll ask, "oh, so you can read my mind right now? What am I thinking?" It may be funny at first, but it does get old after a while.

Many people ask this because as a psychologist or psychology student, you will learn the skills necessary to read human behavior. But mostly this is done through nonverbal communication, body language, and active listening, not mind reading.

26. YOU'LL DO A LOT OF WRITING

If you study psychology, you should be prepared to do a lot of writing. Not only will many of your assignments be research papers, but you may even encounter some essay exams. As a psychologist, you'll also write many reports and notes about your clients. So, writing is part of the program and the career.

27. YOU DON'T ALWAYS NEED THE TEXTBOOK

This tip definitely translates across multiple disciplines and different courses, but you won't always need the textbook. Instead, wait until you are actually in the class before you buy the textbook. If buying the textbook is something you're worried about, you can always ask upperclassmen, the teaching assistants, or even the professor if you have a good relationship with them.

If you do find that your professor requires information from the textbook, you can buy an online version that day or have the textbook in your hands in under a week. In fact, most professors understand that textbooks are expensive and often post the chapters online for all their students to access. So before you drop hundreds of dollars on textbooks, wait to see if you actually need it.

28. GET INTO RESEARCH

If you have the option to get into research, do it. Not only will you gain valuable research experience, but you'll make much better connections with the faculty, students in your major, and even other professors at the university. When working in research at the undergraduate level, you may find positions that are paid and unpaid. While the paid positions are the Holy Grail of research assistantships, you'll get just as much experience working as a volunteer.

You'll learn a lot as an undergrad in research. You'll learn how to do a literature review, how to structure a research project, find participants, learn about ethical review boards, and more. Additionally, you'll also probably get the chance to go to conferences and may even be able to present your research.

Many master's and doctoral programs will look and ask for research experience when you apply. While it is not required for your entrance into a program, having research on your resume or CV may give you an advantage. It can be really difficult to get quality reference letters as well, but researching for a professor will almost guarantee you a fantastic letter of recommendation.

29. SHADOW, SHADOW, SHADOW.

This is something that I did not take as seriously as I should have, and as a result, panicked my senior year trying to figure out what I wanted to do after graduation. So, make sure you pick a couple of jobs in the psychology field that you're interested in and start contacting some people to shadow.

For those who are unfamiliar, shadowing is basically following a professional around for a day to get a sense of what they do for their job. It can be quite beneficial because you'll see what a certain professional does, how they interact with their coworkers, and get a chance to ask them questions about their job.

You should keep in mind, however, that not all professions will allow shadowing. If you are trying to shadow a counselor, for example, you won't be able to sit in on sessions because of confidentiality. In this case, it may be best to interview a counselor instead of shadowing. If you do plan to interview someone, try taking them out for coffee, they usually appreciate that!

When shadowing, you want to explore as many professions as you can, so don't be afraid to shadow multiple people. Even if you are only a bit interested in a profession, check it out! If you know you want to get into psychology, some good jobs to shadow or interview include:

- Occupational Therapists
- Social Workers
- School Psychologists
- Counselors
- Psychiatrists
- Psychological Researchers
- Forensic Psychologists
- Professors (if you're interested in teaching)
- Clinical Psychologists

30. GET TO KNOW YOUR PROFESSORS

Getting to know your professors is great in more ways than one. Reference letters may be one driving factor to visit your professor during office hours. Trying to get a quality reference letter can be hard if you're in a class of over 100 students, so go to office hours and get to know your professors. Not only are you more likely to get reference letters, but if you get to know your professors you may have more opportunities for teaching assistantships, research, and just getting to know a really cool person.

The best ways to get to know your professors are to go to office hours, ask questions about class and their research, and set up appointments to discuss class material. By doing these things, the professors will at least recognize you as you take more advanced courses.

31. WORK ON CAMPUS

Many students opt to work while they are in school, and working can be a great way to pay for tuition, food, and housing without having to take out thousands of dollars worth of loans. However, it can be tricky juggling off-campus work and school. Yes, it can be done, and many students do it, but working on campus is much easier and more convenient.

By working on campus, you can go to class and immediately go to work afterward. Additionally, you usually get much more flexible hours by working on-campus versus off-campus. The downside of working on campus, however, is that you usually only have the option to work part-time. But part-time work does allow you to spend more time focusing on your degree. So really, it's up to you. If you can handle the stress of an off-campus job, go for it. If part-time sounds more your style, then go for one that's on-campus.

32. JOIN PSYCHOLOGY CLUBS

Most universities will have a club specifically for psychology majors. And if they do, join it! Just like in high school, college clubs need to have a professor who sponsors them. Most of the time, that professor is one of the psychology professors. By joining a psychology club, you'll have a better chance of getting closer to your professors.

Additionally, psychology clubs are specifically for psychology majors, so you'll get to meet more students in your major. Not only is it a great opportunity to form study groups, but you may even make some friends at the club meetings and events. Plus, the events are often fun activities that are paid for by the school. Who doesn't want free pizza and a movie night? Join a club and you'll get some!

33. YOU CAN MINOR IN OTHER AREAS

Even if you major in psychology, that doesn't mean you have to only study psychology. In fact, minoring in other areas, such as business, social work, biology, public health or any other area can be an advantage.

With minors in other areas, you can get unique positions, for example:

If you minor in business:
- Advertising Trainee/Agent
- Customer Relations
- Employment Counselor
- Insurance Agent
- Loan Officer
- Marketing Researcher/Representative
- Personnel Administrator
- Public Relations
- Sales Manager

If you get a minor in family and child studies, health-related studies, or sociology:
- Affirmative Action Officer
- Behavioral Analyst
- Community Services Worker
- Counselor
- Day Care Supervisor (children or adults)
- Rehab Advisor
- Social Services Director
- Volunteer Services Director [2]

The biggest thing to keep in mind when choosing a minor is to think about how that minor will affect your goals. If you plan to go into neuroscience, for example, it may be a good idea to minor in biology. But if you know you want to go into forensic psychology, minoring in government or history may be the way to go.

Just make sure to research what you want to do before you make the jump into a minor. Further, your professors or academic advisor can be great resources to help you choose your minor. So, make sure to set up an appointment to talk about your future goals and plans.

34. YOUR MENTAL HEALTH MATTERS

In psychology, you'll hear a lot about coping skills and self-care. While they may seem like you can blow them off and still get by, don't. Your mental health matters as much as your grade, so make sure you take the time you need to de-stress. College is one of the most stressful experiences you'll ever have, and it's absolutely vital that you manage your anxiety, depression, and overall stress.

Some of the best ways to take time to support your mental health are walking, hiking, exercising, sleeping (yes, make sure you're sleeping 8 hours a day), eating healthy, spending time with friends, binging that new series, reading for fun, drawing, journaling, or any other activity that you enjoy.

If you make time for the things you love, you'll be in a much better state of mind and will be able to tackle all the stressful college experiences.

35. YOU'LL READ A LOT

Along with writing, you'll do plenty of reading as a psychology major. Whether it's in the textbook, a new research study, case studies, or an article your professor found interesting, you'll be doing a lot of reading. This is especially true in the field of psychology, so be prepared.

An important part of reading—and an absolutely necessary skill—is being able to skim. Skimming means you read the most important parts of the reading, but don't go too in-depth. Basically, you need the major points, the results, and any important implications of the reading. If you can write down 3 to 5 talking points, you should be golden.

If you try to read everything in-depth and take super detailed notes, you'll end up being burnt out and spend hours on each reading assignment. Of course, it's all important information, but you can skim to get the highlights and be just fine.

36. STUDY ABROAD

If you have the opportunity to study abroad, take it! Studying abroad is a great way to see the world, learn about a different culture, and see how psychology is implemented in different parts of the world. Many universities offer programs for study abroad, and there are generally two types.

With one, you'll go with an entire group of students to study abroad in a different country, such as Ireland, Italy, or Peru. These trips may be for an entire semester, but they may also be for a month over winter or summer break. This type of study abroad may be good for students who don't want to go overseas alone or who don't need to go for an entire semester but still want to travel.

The other type of study abroad is where you stay with a host family for an entire semester or year. Instead of going with a group of students from your school, you attend a new school and take their classes. This type of study abroad is definitely more adventurous but can be one of the most amazing experiences.

If you know you want to study abroad, make sure your advisor knows early on in your academic career. You can plan when you will study abroad as early as your freshmen year. That way, you won't run into the problem of not having enough credits to graduate in the typical four years.

37. JOIN PROFESSIONAL ORGANIZATIONS

Professional organizations in psychology offer many awesome benefits. As a student, you don't have to pay as much for a membership as working professionals, so you can get access to conferences, new research, textbooks, professional developments, forums, and more for a cheaper price.

As a college student, the American Psychological Association (APA) may be one of the best options for you to join, but if you're interested in a certain area of psychology, you can join more specific professional organizations. In fact, you don't need to limit yourself to just one organization; you can join many!

For example, you could join:
- American Psychological Association
- Graduate Students in APA
- American Educational Research Association (AERA)
- Association for Psychological Science (APS)
- Junior Researchers in EARLI (JURE)
- Society for Personality and Social Psychology (SPSP)
- National Association for Multicultural Education (NAME)
- School Psychologist Professional Organizations
- American Psychological Association
- National Association of School Psychologists
- Counseling Psychologist Professional Associations
- American Psychological Association
- APA Division 35 (Society for the Psychology of Women)
- National Black Counseling Psychologists
- Association of Black Psychologists [3]

38. LEARNING BEYOND THE CLASSROOM: GET AN INTERNSHIP

Internships can be great experiences and look incredible on a resume. With an internship, you'll practice your psychology skills and learn what psychology looks like in practice. Most of the time, you can only get an internship in your Junior or Senior year, but sometimes Sophomores or Freshmen can get internships.

Internships are jobs that typically take place over the summer. However, some psychology programs require an internship, and it will take place during the semester. In some cases, you will get paid for your work; in other cases, you don't get paid but will get college credit. Regardless of how you do your internship, they are worth it.

However, having an internship will not make or break your psychology career. While it may look good, you can still be successful without one. So, don't fret if you don't have many opportunities or need to continue working at a current job to support yourself.

50 Things to Know

PSYCHOLOGY SKILLS AND MORE

Many of your psychology skills will become developed throughout your studies, but in this section, we'll cover some of the key skills that you will need in order to succeed in the psychology field.

39. REFLECTION IS KEY TO THE PSYCH DEGREE

A major part of studying psychology is reflection. You'll learn how to help your clients to reflect, and the best way to learn is to become a master reflector yourself. Oftentimes, you do reflection exercises and assignments that ask you to reflect on classwork, readings, and other activities. By the time you are done with your psychology degree, you'll be reflecting on your work in psychology, but also nearly everything else.

40. THE IMPORTANCE OF COUNSELING MICRO SKILLS

Counseling micros kills are your basic tools for creating good counseling relationships. You will learn to use micros kills to build rapport, create an empathetic relationship, and promote genuineness, acceptance, and understanding. These skills are the foundation of your practice, and will include:

- Eye contact
- Validation
- Non-verbal body language
- Tone of voice
- Active listening
- Open and closed questions
- Paraphrasing
- Summarizing
- Reflecting

You'll learn how to incorporate these skills in your practice and will spend a lot of time studying them. If you get to know them now, you'll already be ahead of the crowd! [4]

41. "TELL ME MORE"

You'll find yourself saying this to clients all the time. Why, do you ask? Because it is the number one phrase that will get your client to literally tell you more about something they might not want to talk about. "Tell me more" will be one of your best open-ended questions to use in your toolkit of micro skills. Not only will you use the phrase for class, but you'll find yourself using it in everyday conversations as well.

So if you use this phrase in one of your entry-level psychology classes, you'll absolutely knock the socks off your professor and look like a pro.

42. ACCEPT CONSTRUCTIVE CRITICISM

Feedback and constructive criticism are a given in the psych field. Some people enjoy getting feedback because it helps them improve their work, but most people will find that accepting feedback can be hard at first. This is because some feedback—especially if you are in advanced courses or programs—can be harsh. You may put hours into an assignment and think it was perfect, but then get a ton of not-so-nice feedback that you weren't expecting.

But keep in mind that feedback and constructive criticism are good things. The alternative would be that you get a poor grade and have no idea why. Additionally, accepting criticism and incorporating it into your work can only make you a better student and professional.

If you have the mindset that feedback will help you improve, you'll be more likely to look for feedback. While some professors will provide excess feedback, others will ask you to come to their office to discuss your paper or assignment. Remember, you can really get to know your professor if you spend time discussing assignments, so use feedback as an opportunity!

43. GET ALONG WITH OTHERS

While being good with people is virtually a given if you want to work in human and social services, it's still important to mention. To be successful in the field of psychology, you will need to have solid people skills and want to work with people. In most positions, you will work with people every day whether they be clients or coworkers.

This doesn't mean that you need to be an extrovert, it just means that you should know that most of your job requires interacting with people. Some jobs will require less human interaction, such as research, but you will still need to work with people daily even if you aren't counseling all day.

Even if you are an introvert (like I am), you should still have a passion for helping people and want a job that requires you to interact with people. The most important skills are simply good listening, the ability to read body language, and the ability to form healthy relationships and boundaries. If you can do all these things, you can work with people as a psychological professional.

44. PSYCH JOBS ARE NOT EASY

Many people think that psychology jobs are easy because all you do is talk to people all day. Well, that's not the case. Even if you're a counselor who specializes in telehealth, you will be tired and encounter a great deal of stress.

As a counselor, you will see clients, write reports, and plan interventions for your clients. Your entire day will be busy, and the work can be stressful. You'll have easy clients, but you'll also have challenging clients that require you to research and prepare for your sessions. This is especially true for new therapists because they don't have the practical experience to jump into a session. Instead, you'll be thinking about which counseling micro skill you should use and why.

Additionally, active listening requires a lot of work. You need to be paying full attention to what the client is saying so that you can reflect with them, make connections to what they said earlier, paraphrase, or come up with the perfect question to guide the conversation.

While many counselors do take notes during their sessions, notetaking can actually damage the relationship with your client because they think you aren't paying attention. So, you need to work really hard to take as few notes as possible but still remember everything that happened in the session.

The jobs in psychology can be especially difficult if you have experienced similar mental health challenges. It's fairly common for those who have struggled with mental health to go into the psychology field. It can be a strength to know what the client may be experiencing, but it can also be triggering for the therapist. This is why copings skills and stress management are so important. I've said it before, and I'll say it again: always keep your own mental health in mind when you work in the psychology field.

45. PERSONAL GROWTH

Finally, personal growth is essential to working in the psychology field. When you begin to learn about psychology, counseling, and theories, you'll begin to learn a lot about who you are as a person and make connections that you never thought about.

But personal growth will only happen if you remain open-minded. You can remain rigid in your old ways and habits, but this will not help you grow as a psychology professional. Those who work in psychology are always looking for ways to expand their knowledge and expertise, so if you are not willing to do that, psychology may not be the field for you.

AFTER YOUR DEGREE

Whether you've just completed your bachelor's degree or have recently defended your doctoral level dissertation, there are some things that you should be prepared for after you graduate with your psychology degree.

As you now know, there are many jobs in psychology besides counseling. You have the option to get into cutting-edge research, work in neuroscience, or even study human behavior. The opportunities are endless! But how do you specialize and what can you do with those specializations? In this section, we'll look at psychology licensure and where you can specialize in your career as a psychologist or psychological professional.

46. YOU CAN ONLY BE LICENSED WITH A GRADUATE DEGREE

To become a licensed psychologist, you need to get licensed through your state's licensing board. The first step to becoming licensed is to get a master's, specialist, or doctoral degree in your field of choice. Keep in mind that different areas require different levels of licensing. For example, you generally need a specialist degree in school psychology, but you will need a doctoral degree to become a clinical psychologist.

Typically, you will need to get a graduate-level degree, get around 2,000 hours of professional supervision, pass your Praxis or Examination for Professional Practice in Psychology, pass a state licensing exam, and then become a licensed psychologist. [5]

47. LICENSES DON'T ALWAYS TRANSER FROM STATE TO STATE

Just because you have a license in Minnesota does not mean you'll have a license in California. This is because the license requirements vary from state to state. Some states require different testing, others don't require a license to practice in a certain area, and some require a separate degree to practice. The best way to figure out what your state requires for licensing is to look at your state's website for psychology licensure. Usually, the process of transferring your license to a different state is tedious, but it can be done.

You should always review your state's licensing requirements before you attend a program. Why? Because not all programs have the qualifications for every state. When you look for a program, you want to find one that is accredited by APA because those programs will be more likely to transfer. If you still are not sure, try talking to professors or academic advisors to see if students have been licensed in the state you wish to practice.

48. SEPARATE WORK FROM HOME

Separating work from home is easier said than done. In any job that requires working with people, you'll encounter some situations that are difficult to let go of. With any situation that involves trauma, working with historically marginalized populations, or working with those who are suffering, you will need some time to process.

That being said, you'll need to develop a healthy work and life balance. You'll need to use your coping skills and stress management skills to help you process the events of your day so that you can go home and leave work behind. While this may sound easy or at least doable, there will be some days that your mind will be at work and your body at home. You'll overthink something you said, wish you had tried something different, or maybe just wish something had gone differently.

Now, these are all perfectly normal things to think about. But keep them at work. Otherwise, you risk burning out of your job and find yourself thinking about work more than you do the activities you love. For some people, they aim to forget the workday the second they leave their office. Others, such as myself, find that processing the workday while driving home is the best way to think about the day and let it go.

Regardless of how you do it, you need to find a way to leave work at work so that you can enjoy your home life. If you find yourself struggling with this, try talking to your colleagues, mentors, coworkers, or another professional counselor for tips and tricks.

49. YOU CAN SPECIALIZE

There are so many jobs in psychology beyond counseling. As you're working towards your degree in psychology, you should also reflect on the areas that you find fascinating. After all, this is the career that you will likely be doing until you retire, so you should make sure it's in an area that you are passionate about! While new areas of psychology are popping up all over the place (like positive psychology, the study of happiness and positive traits), you can specialize in the areas below.

Counseling Psychology. This is probably what most people fall back on when they think about a career in psychology. Those who enter the field of counseling help clients deal with issues regarding adjustment to changes in their lives as well as various mental health problems, such as anxiety, depression, suicidal ideation, eating disorders, addiction, and more. Counseling psychologists generally work in clinics, agencies, or directly with individuals in private practice.

Even though counseling psychology can be considered a specialization all its own, it's also important to note that you can specialize in areas of counseling as well. For example, you could become a marriage counselor, addictions counselor, school counselor, or child counselor. Mostly, those who pursue counseling will choose a population (group of people) that they prefer to work with.

Environmental Psychology. Environmental psychologists are mainly tasked with creating environments that promote successful living. Oftentimes, they work to make physical settings comfortable and functional for all populations. Generally, environmental psychologists will work with architects, urban or city planners, and may even work with biologists and conservationists in natural environments.

Health Psychology. Professionals in health psychology work to promote health education in communities. They may also diagnose, assign treatment, and work on projects that aim to support the prevention of illness. Additionally, health psychologists may help people in their communities change their attitudes about risk-related behaviors that are commonly associated with poor health, such as smoking, unprotected sex, and obesity.

Educational Psychology. Those who work in educational psychology or school psychology research better learning and teacher techniques to better support children in the schools. Moreover, educational psychologists will apply their knowledge to enhance school curriculum and instruction. Educational psychologists typically work directly with students, educators, administrators, and businesses that provide education.

Media Psychology. Professionals working in media psychology research how electronic and printed information (such as social media platforms) affects individuals, especially children and adolescents who are influenced by today's television and online media. Typically, media psychologists are work in journalism, broadcasting, and education and will assist media personnel in developing formats that deliver positive messages.

Legal Psychology. Legal psychologists use psychological practices and theories to improve laws and help individuals better understand the complex legal system. As a legal psychologist, you may work with groups of people by educating them on the court process. Some people in legal psychology may also evaluate convicted individuals if their mental health is in question.

Abnormal Psychology. Abnormal psychologists study the science of mental illness, the causes, and treatments of mental disorders. Many individuals who go into the field of abnormal psychology work in the medical field as researchers and will need rather intense postgraduate studies and specialization.

Clinical Psychology. Clinical psychologists mainly diagnose and treat mental disorders. They typically provide counseling services, conduct research studies, and may teach at the post-secondary level. To become a clinical psychologist, you'll need five years of graduate study and a year-long internship to earn a doctorate.

Psychiatry. As you found out in the previous sections, psychiatrists are medical doctors who specialize in the diagnosis and treatment of mental illness. They often prescribe medication and will sometimes provide treatment, but will mostly focus on prescriptions.

Social Work. Instead of treating mental illness, social workers are more concerned with the social and cultural aspects of human behavior. Social workers will work in a variety of settings, such as schools, hospitals, social services agencies, courts, and prisons. [2]

50. BE YOUR OWN BOSS

If you receive your doctorate degree and have a few years of experience in the psychology field, you can open your own practice and run your very own psychology clinic. While there are many pros and cons to doing so, the opportunity to work as the head of your own practice may seem very tempting to some in the field of psychology.

Running a private practice can be incredibly rewarding because it allows you to set your own hours and makes your career much more flexible. While some psychologists go as far as to have their own physical practice in a business building, others are finding that telehealth is a great way to privately practice. With telehealth, you can be your own psychologist and simply pay for the online platform. Additionally, many online telehealth services advertise for you, so getting clients doesn't have to be difficult.

If opening a private practice is your goal, then you may want to work in private practice to gain experience and insight into what it will be like. For many people, figuring out billing and accepting clients' insurance is the most difficult part of owning a practice. However, if you take some business management and health information systems courses in college or after you've gotten your psychology degree, you'll be prepared to run your own practice.

Should you be interested in opening a private practice or becoming a consultant, make sure you make your goals known to any graduate school advisors as they often have great resources and expert advice that can get you to where you need to be.

FINAL THOUGHTS

As you can see, there is a lot to know about the psychology degree. Now that you know about psychology as a science, the history of the field, what jobs you can pursue, and tips for college success, you'll be ready to start your path as a psychology major.

As you're studying psychology, it's important to remember that this field will require a lot of self-evaluation and reflection. Not only will you learn about how to help others, but you'll be challenged by tasks that require you to think about who you are, where you came from, and how your life experiences will influence your practice.

Not only will you learn a lot about yourself, but you'll be in a position to make positive changes and great impacts in the lives of others. With a psychology degree, you're a master of mental health and a person who knows how to expertly work with people and actively listen. You can use these skills in your professional life, but don't be afraid to utilize your psychology skills in other aspects of life too, you may find that your relationships with family and friends become better because of it. But never forget that ever-so-important work-life balance, you'll thank me later.

As you begin your psychological studies, you should remember to refer back to the sections in this book that apply to your needs, especially if you are trying to decide whether you want to pursue higher education or specialize in a certain area of psychology. And more than anything, share what you know about the psychology field with your peers and classmates because you're now a master of everything psychology.

OTHER RESOURCES:

1. https://psychology.ucdavis.edu/research/research-areas#:~:text=The%20UC%20Davis%20Department%20of,take%20seminars%20in%20all%20five.

2. https://www.mycollegeoptions.org/content/research/major/Description/Psychology.aspx

3. http://www.psychologist-license.com/types-of-psychologists/psychologist-associations/

4. https://www.sulross.edu/sites/default/files/sites/default/files/users/docs/education/counseling-microskills_4.pdf

5. https://www.apa.org/gradpsych/2004/01/get-licensed

6. https://www.psychologydegree411.com/careers/#assoc

7. https://www.apa.org/ed/precollege/psn/2018/01/bachelors-degree

8. https://www.apa.org/ed/precollege/psn/2017/01/masters-careers

9. https://www.waldenu.edu/online-doctoral-programs/phd-in-psychology/resource/what-can-you-do-with-a-phd-in-psychology

10. https://www.bls.gov/ooh/life-physical-and-social-science/psychologists.htm#tab-6

11. https://www.apa.org/monitor/2008/06/undergrad-major
12. http://personal.psu.edu/faculty/a/c/acp103/PSYCH105/brief_history.htm
13. https://www.simplypsychology.org/Sigmund-Freud.html

OTHER HELPFUL RESOURCES

For more information about psychology and degrees, check out these resources.

- The American Psychological Association
  https://www.apa.org/
-
- College Navigator Tool
  https://nces.ed.gov/collegenavigator/
-
- US Bureau of Labor Statistics
  https://www.bls.gov/

READ OTHER 50 THINGS TO KNOW BOOKS

50 Things to Know About Coping With Stress: By A Mental Health Specialist by Kimberly L. Brownridge

50 Things to Know About Being a Zookeeper: Life of a Zookeeper by Stephanie Fowlie

50 Things to Know About Becoming a Doctor: The Journey from Medical School of the Medical Profession by Tong Liu MD

50 Things to Know About Knitting: Knit, Purl, Tricks & Shortcuts by Christina Fanelli

50 Things to Know

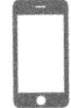

Stay up to date with new releases on Amazon:
https://amzn.to/2VPNGr7

CZYKPublishing.com

50 Things to Know

We'd love to hear what you think about our content! Please leave your honest review of this book on Amazon and Goodreads. We appreciate your positive and constructive feedback. Thank you.

50 THINGS TO KNOW BOOK SERIES REVIEWS FROM READERS

I recently downloaded a couple of books from this series to read over the weekend thinking I would read just one or two. However, I so loved the books that I read all the six books I had downloaded in one go and ended up downloading a few more today. Written by different authors, the books offer practical advice on how you can perform or achieve certain goals in life, which in this case is how to have a better life.

The information is simple to digest and learn from, and is incredibly useful. There are also resources listed at the end of the book that you can use to get more information.

50 Things To Know To Have A Better Life: Self-Improvement Made Easy!

Author Dannii Cohen

This book is very helpful and provides simple tips on how to improve your everyday life. I found it to be useful in improving my overall attitude.

50 Things to Know For Your Mindfulness & Meditation Journey
Author Nina Edmondso

Quick read with 50 short and easy tips for what to think about before starting to homeschool.

50 Things to Know About Getting Started with Homeschool by Author Amanda Walton

i

I really enjoyed the voice of the narrator, she speaks in a soothing tone. The book is a really great reminder of things we might have known we could do during stressful times, but forgot over the years.

Author Harmony Hawaii

There is so much waste in our society today. Everyone should be forced to read this book. I know I am passing it on to my family.

50 Things to Know to Downsize Your Life: How To Downsize, Organize, And Get Back to Basics

Author Lisa Rusczyk Ed. D.

Great book to get you motivated and understand why you may be losing motivation. Great for that person who wants to start getting healthy, or just for you when you need motivation while having an established workout routine.

50 Things To Know To Stick With A Workout: Motivational Tips To Start The New You Today

Author Sarah Hughes